THE
RESILIENCE RESET

A Woman's Journey Through Medical
Challenges And The Search For Answers
To Reclaim Health And Joy

JOSETTE MANDELA

The Resilience Reset

Copyright @ 2024 by Josette Mandela

Disclaimer Notice

Please note the information contained in this document is for educational and entertainment purposes. All effort has been made to present accurate, reliable, and complete information. No warranties of any kind are declared or implied. Readers acknowledge the author does not render legal, financial, medical or professional advice. The content within this book is from various sources. Readers are encouraged to consult with relevant experts or authorities in specific fields for advice and guidance.

By reading this book, the reader agrees that under no circumstances is the author or publisher responsible for any direct or indirect losses incurred due to the use of the information contained within.

First published by Brindled Butterfly Investments, Inc.

1015 Atlantic Blvd, Suite 402

Atlantic Beach, FL 32233

ISBN: 978-1-7348771-4-4 - hardcover
ISBN: 978-1-7348771-2-0 - paperbook
ISBN: 978-1-7348771-3-7 - ebook
ISBN: 978-1-7348771-5-1 - audiobook
Library of Congress Control Number: 2024905798

My way of saying Thank you.

I appreciate your taking the time to read this book. I created this free resource with useful tips to help you on your journey.

To download the free bonus material for this book, please visit:

https://www.TheResilienceResetBook.com/bonus

Contents

Chapter One: Is this my life?   1

Chapter Two: Off to college   5

Chapter Three: The drama begins   9

Chapter Four: Time goes on   13

Chapter Five: The rest of the story   27

Chapter Six: And then…   39

Chapter Seven: Dream Life   43

Chapter Eight: Yet more tests   49

Chapter Nine: Now what   61

Chapter Ten: It's up to Me   65

Chapter Eleven: Your gifts   69

Chapter Twelve: A new beginning   73

About the Author   77

Chapter One

Is this my life?

I magine lying curled up in a ball on the floor. You're whimpering like a scared puppy, holding your head in your hands, hoping someone—anyone—can put an end to this excruciating pain in your left ear.

Then imagine trying to get off the floor. As you move, you're hit with a blinding migraine, nausea, and the feeling the world is spinning out of control. You crawl to the bathroom and hug the toilet. Since you haven't eaten for eighteen hours, your stomach is empty. The waves of nausea erupt in dry heaves.

You spend twenty minutes like this. When the nausea gets less intense; you crawl to the couch and try to sleep.

This is where the journey gets real. But how did I get here? What led up to this situation?

In the beginning

Imagine a gentle, babbling brook, surrounded by children at play, their laughter mingling with the sound of water. On this warm, sunny summer day, time stretches endlessly before them. Sunlight filters through the trees, casting a lazy dance on the water's surface, occasionally birthing rainbows. It's an idyllic snapshot in time."

This scene vividly recalls my childhood, when my sister and I would venture into the woods behind our house to play by a stream we discovered. We gave the small island in the middle of the stream a name, Namboombu, from the movie *Bedknobs and Broomsticks*. We had hours of fun, jumping from the side of the stream to the "island" and back. Some days we would walk upstream, looking for the start of the headwater, other days we'd walk downstream curious where it might have ended.

That was a time when everything seemed possible. The adventure, the thrill of doing something just because it was fun and not because you had to. I could be a doctor, lawyer, race car driver, anything was possible. There were no expectations, no worries, no thoughts about if it would even be possible.

Back then, ideas came 'fast and furious.' One day, I wanted to be a doctor and heal the sick, the next a race car driver and have fame and fortune by being the fastest on the track. Another day, I want to be a plumber like my uncle.

As a child, dreams know no bounds. Youth unveils a world of endless possibilities, each one a viable option, a potential path. Why couldn't I envision myself as a doctor, a race car driver, or an animal trainer?

Then you become an *adult* and everything changes.

High school presented a unique chapter in my life, growing up in a town so small it lacked its own high school. Connecticut offered me two choices: attend the public high school in the neighboring town or embark on a longer journey to the vocational agricultural high school three towns away.

My mother treated finding a high school the same way most people treat going to college. She made appointments at the two schools the state would pay for, and added a nearby Catholic high school as well. Each school we visited had a class schedule for me to follow.

These were my choices, for better or worse. The town provided bus service to both the public high school and the vocational agricultural school, a crucial service since both of my parents worked and we lived in a rural area. Commuting by school bus or carpool was our only option. More importantly, both schools were publicly funded, covered by state and local taxes, ensuring there was no cost to attend.

Additionally, my mother considered a Catholic school that was a mere five-minute drive from our home. Given our Catholic faith, this was her preferred choice for my education, despite the financial commitment required to enroll me there.

The public high school was a mess. Students constantly disrespected the teacher and nobody paid attention in class. It was chaos. The Catholic school was the opposite extreme. Everyone was respectful. Unfortunately, the curriculum was four years of French and did not include calculus. I had already taken one year of Spanish and Algebra 1. I did not want to start with a new language and also did not want to repeat Algebra 1. So to me, both choices were off the table.

Finally, we visited the vocational agricultural high school, and it was a happy medium. I could take calculus my senior year, and I had the choice of either Spanish or French as a foreign language. The agricultural school offered a mix of respectful students and class clowns; however, the teachers took better control of the classroom so there was no chaos. Students who misbehaved were sent to the principal's office to maintain a serene learning environment. This was a sharp contrast to the public school I had visited.

While in high school, I joined a medical explorer post. Explorer posts are a co-ed arm of the Boy Scouts of America organization for children too old to attend either sect of scouts. A perk of being a member of the medical explorer post was access to the local hospital and the possibility of getting a scholarship to study to become an emergency medical technician (EMT). At sixteen, I was not only one of the youngest students in the EMT program; I was also one of the youngest to complete the program.

Chapter Exercises

Take fifteen minutes to ponder your current choices.

Do you act like every day is fun and a new adventure is waiting for you around every corner?

Or are you more like I was? Putting on my business suit most days and leaving fun and adventure for weekends. Or maybe you find you need to work the weekends too, so fun gets relegated to vacations and maybe holidays?

Which life would you rather have?

Do you want to keep the life you have now where everything seems difficult and nothing is fun? Or is now the time to reconnect with that childlike wonder?

After you have really thought about your choices, journal about the experience. How did it feel to add childlike wonder back into your life?

Chapter Two

Off to college

In the '70s, most families wanted their children to go to college. A college degree could mean a difference of $5,000 or more to your initial salary. Back then, parents often pushed their children toward college, sometimes against their will. Fortunately, the saving grace was the abundance of affordable options available at that time. There were colleges to fit most pocketbooks, eliminating the need for large loans to get a degree; community colleges, small private religious-based schools, even technical colleges were feasible.

Drawn by my ambition to become a medical doctor, I opted for a school renowned for its exemplary science program. I was even awarded an honor scholarship that covered half of the tuition fees. The sole condition for retaining this scholarship was maintaining a grade-point average of 3.0.

Four years later, I graduated from college with a bachelor's degree in Biochemistry. I soon realized having barely passed the medical entrance exam (MCAT) and not having rich parents, I would not be going to medical school.

I was mad about this unfair situation, and after some deep reflection decided that there must be something else I was put on this earth to do. Though I really enjoyed working in the medical field, I decided to let that dream go. I took the rejection in stride and chose to look at other options.

Several classmates were working at Yale University, and I decided to join them as a lab technician.

I landed a position at the Human Genetics lab and was excited to be involved in groundbreaking research, helping to cure devastating diseases. One disease being studied in our lab was Tay Sachs' disease. It is a terminal illness that affects Jewish children. The scientists in the lab were studying and theorizing about various diseases and how to cure them. They were also very secretive about what they did and knew. The more questions I asked, the less they wanted to share.

That was when I learned about the 'publish or perish' mantra of the academic world.

This implies that failing to publish an article within a designated timeframe could render both you and your research obsolete. Even more daunting is the possibility that another researcher might solve the question you've dedicated yourself to answering.

This revelation was completely unexpected. I had harbored the naive belief that the scientific community was united in a collective pursuit for the common good. The reality, however, was starkly different: the competition was cutthroat, and the prevailing secrecy among researchers was startling. This point was driven home after I had been working at the lab for about one week. One of my friends from college worked in a different lab and invited me to lunch. I was excited to tell her about the things I'd been doing since college and find out how her life was going.

Imagine my surprise when I came back from lunch and was accosted by several senior-level members of my lab. Why did you go to lunch with someone from that lab? What did they ask you? What did you tell them about what we are doing? On and on their questions went!

My answers were essentially that I went to lunch with a college friend. We talked about what we've been doing since college. We did not discuss work as we haven't seen each other since graduation. There was plenty to talk about besides work....

The whole incident made me question my life choices and whether I could have a career as a lab technician. After a few more weeks of equally invasive and disrespectful behavior, I decided that working in this lab was not a good fit for me.

In order to pursue a different career, I needed a different degree. I researched the local colleges for inspiration. I was sure that to get a job in the corporate world, I would need a Master of Business Administration(MBA). Doing that research, I discovered a nearby college was offering a dual degree program in the same amount of time that other schools granted an MBA.

As I wasn't sure where I was going next, I decided having two masters could help me find something I wanted to pursue as a career. That convinced me to pursue the dual degree program at the University of New Haven. I felt disappointed that my first career choice had not worked out, but was excited about my next adventure.

To support my education, I secured a job at a local bank, which offered the flexibility necessary to manage both full-time work and college studies. Looking back, I am equally amazed at my health and fitness during that period. In my twenties and thirties, maintaining my health or weight seemed effortless, a fact that often sparked envy among peers.

At buffets, I could indulge in everything at least once without gaining weight, a feat that delighted me. Yet, what many didn't realize was that such indulgences were the exception, not the rule, in my diet. I adhered to a Spartan regimen, consuming what some might consider barely enough calories to sustain a bird. But coupled with regular exercise, this lifestyle suited me perfectly. Whether compensating for a day's feast with a rigorous session at the gym, a leisurely walk in my neighborhood, or a run on the beach, I managed to balance it all. Reflecting on those times, I can't help but cherish the vibrancy of my life then.

Chapter Exercise:

Take fifteen minutes to journal about the following statements.

Think about what you wanted to be when you grew up. Write down what that life looked like.

If that is not your life, write down where you are today and how you feel about being here.

Chapter Three

The drama begins

After two and a half years of dedicated study, I emerged with two master's degrees, poised to embark on the next chapter of my life. Armed with a Master of Business Administration (MBA), I hoped this accomplishment would suffice, allowing me to step away from the academic world. My desire was to forge ahead with my life beyond the confines of college, eager to explore what lay outside the realm of academia.

After distributing fifty resumes in response to newspaper advertisements, I secured a few interviews. One particularly promising offer came from a software company. Despite lacking the specific background they typically sought, the company's lead technical expert recognized the value of my diverse experience. My tenure as a teller, culminating in the role of assistant branch manager over three and a half years, demonstrated my capability in handling customer service issues effectively without causing upset. Moreover, my academic achievements underscored a consistent dedication: if I committed to a task, I would see it through to completion.

That conversation has stuck with me my whole life. I always want to be the person people can rely on. When I say I am going to do something, I do it.

Before embarking on this new career journey, my boyfriend and I decided to escape for a weekend getaway in upstate New York, just a short drive from where we lived. On our second day, while waiting at a left turn lane for the green light, a moment of alarm gripped us as a truck barreled through the red light on our right. We barely had time to sigh in relief at our narrow escape when suddenly—WHAM—a collision thrust us into the middle of the intersection.

The 65-year-old man driving a large sedan saw the pickup go through the light and, not paying attention, plowed into the back of our car at sixty miles per hour. That is what the official police report stated. This event occurred before headrests were required in passenger vehicles. Having a long neck, I immediately knew I was hurt. My neck felt like it wouldn't support my head and my back was on fire. When the police arrived, they called for an ambulance, which then took me to the emergency room.

Once there, the doctor ordered x-rays of my neck and spine. It was determined I had the worst case of whiplash he had ever seen.

Two days later, I started my new job. I was in pain and wearing both a neck and back brace to work. Fortunately, I have a high tolerance for pain and survived the day. The president of the company offered me a recommendation to an orthopedic surgeon, so I made an appointment for a couple of days later.

After we talked about my x-rays and how I was feeling, the doctor wrote a prescription for painkillers (800 mg Motrin) and set me up with six months of physical therapy. Therapy consisted of warm, wet blankets to loosen the muscles in my back and light massage for my neck muscles.

The physical therapist also gave me a handout showing some gentle stretching exercises I could do at home. They included neck circles, hip circles, and touching my toes, both standing and sitting on the floor.

After six months of regular visits to the therapist, I went to see the orthopedic surgeon for a follow-up appointment. I asked, "Where do we go from here? Things seem to have hit a plateau. Is this as good as it gets?"

The reply was astonishing. He said, "If you were older, I would recommend surgery. However, as you are still in your twenties, I do not recommend that option."

He outlined a sobering standard within the field: roughly every ten years post-surgery, additional back surgery becomes necessary. This timeframe varies—some extend beyond it, while others face complications that demand earlier intervention. On average, a decade marks the span between interventions in back surgery.

Hearing this was refreshing, yet daunting. The physician's candid admission—that his expertise could, in the long term, introduce further complications rather than resolve them—was a stark revelation. 'Sorry, there's nothing more I can do for you. My training, though well-intentioned, may only lead to more challenges for you down the line,' he seemed to say. Taking his advice to heart, I chose to endure the pain, all the while continuing my quest for alternative solutions to my condition.

Chapter Exercise:

Spend fifteen minutes journaling about your own current health situation.

If you are healthy with no health challenges, congratulations! Journal about what you are doing now and will continue to do in the future to maintain your health.

If you have health challenges:

Do you have a chronic illness or a temporary health challenge?

Have you given up on doing certain activities you love because of chronic pain?

Are you taking multiple prescriptions?

These yes/no questions are just suggestions for areas to review. Maybe you have allergies and routinely see your doctor for shots. Or you go out somewhere, someone sneezes, and you end up sick!

I know we like to think, *The doctor has all this training and knowledge so he must know better than me.* The fact is the more information you gather about your condition and share with your doctor, the more likely the doctor will be to find a solution to your issue(s).

So don't skip this exercise. Put some thought into where you are now and where you want to be physically. You can't build a plan to reach your goal if you don't have a health goal.

This research is not meant to bypass going to the doctor for your condition, this exercise is meant to make you a better-informed patient. There is a lot of new research being done every day. Your doctor may not be able to keep up with all the new breakthroughs that occur so it is up to you to advocate for yourself.

Chapter Four

Time goes on

In my quest for answers, I encountered individuals who had turned to alternative healthcare practitioners for relief. Their experiences opened my eyes to the potential of chiropractors, nutritionists, and other non-traditional health professionals. A chiropractor was able to adjust my spine, significantly reducing my discomfort. Nutritionists, equipped with a range of diagnostic tests, offered a forum to discuss my symptoms. Together, we explored theories that might explain the root cause of my issues.

Upon consulting a nutritionist, they would arrange tests to validate their hypotheses before recommending dietary adjustments and lifestyle modifications aimed at alleviating symptoms. This approach introduced me to a way of life that wasn't dominated by the severe whiplash I endured, nor by the continuous use of pain medication. Additionally, I discovered the benefits of regular exercise in keeping my muscles and joints supple, which, in turn, minimized the inflammation and swelling in my back and neck.

The nutritionist's tests pinpointed specific foods that triggered inflammatory reactions in my body, advising me to avoid them. Surprisingly, many of these foods were ones I didn't particularly enjoy, making them easier to eliminate from my diet. However, cucumbers, despite my confusion over their inclusion, were also recommended for exclusion. Trusting the professional advice, I complied and removed them from my diet.

Gradually, I found it possible to reintroduce some of these foods in moderation. Yet, overconsumption or frequent ingestion led to adverse reactions, varying from mild discomfort to severe migraines. The unpredictability of these outcomes taught me the importance of adhering closely to the prescribed dietary regimen.

Reflecting on the aftermath of the car accident, I remembered how medical professionals had initially listed activities I should avoid to manage my injury. However, two decades later, advancements in research and treatment methodologies offered new perspectives on managing whiplash. With caution, I began incorporating these innovative approaches into my daily routine, seeking a balance between traditional wisdom and contemporary practices.

This journey from conventional medical advice to exploring alternative healthcare solutions underscored a broader lesson about the dynamic nature of health management. It highlighted the value of being open to change while carefully considering new information and practices, especially when dealing with chronic conditions or injuries.

Sprained Instep

Fast forward another twenty years, and I found myself dealing with a sprained instep for what felt like the thousandth time—a statement that might seem like hyperbole but is grounded in a peculiar reality. At the tender age of six, I was diagnosed with extra bones in my feet, an anomaly that rendered my insteps particularly vulnerable. This anatomical quirk meant that any careless step could lead to a painful sprain.

As a child, heedless of these limitations, I engaged fully in running, jumping, and playing. This often resulted in turning too swiftly or landing too harshly, inevitably leading to a sprained instep. Such incidents frequently culminated in visits to the emergency room. After numerous such episodes—whether it was the tenth or the twentieth—I resolved to spare my mother the hassle and manage the situation on my own.

By then, I was well-versed in the necessary steps for recovery, succinctly summarized by the acronym RICE: rest, ice, compression, and elevation. Following a couple of days dedicated to these measures, heat therapy would become beneficial. For compression, an ace bandage was the tool of choice, and my collection of them had grown with each visit to the emergency room. I had accumulated enough to navigate my recovery independently, applying the lessons learned from those repeated visits.

In my 40s, I took a job as a consultant and traveled a lot for work, but I still went to the gym every day. There wasn't much else to do after dark when you're a consultant. After work, especially when away from home and family, the gym offered a productive way to fill the evenings that otherwise had limited options for activities.

However, the challenge of maintaining weight while on the road became apparent. The caloric density and nutritional shortcomings of restaurant meals gradually led to weight gain. Initially, the change was barely noticeable, but by the age of forty-eight, I found myself carrying an extra fifty pounds on my 5-foot-8-inch frame. Despite my dissatisfaction with this development, the solution eluded me. Transitioning out of consulting back to a conventional nine-to-five job did not immediately remedy the situation. It took me some time to realize that I had inadvertently given up my exercise routine amidst the change. On the brighter side, the new job allowed me to adopt a regular eating schedule, facilitating healthier, well-balanced meals. Yet, the absence of physical activity meant that the weight remained, a stark reminder of the need for a balanced approach to health that includes both diet and exercise..

And then I heard about a 10,000-step-a-day challenge. I can't remember whether it was the American Heart Association program or the new Fitbit app, but I joined in with gusto.

Initially, the idea of walking 10,000 steps daily appeared daunting. However, this perspective shifted after I invested in a Fitbit. To my surprise, achieving this goal was more feasible than I had anticipated. The routine journey from my car in the parking lot to my desk, coupled with the incidental strolls around the office throughout the day, and then back to my car, amounted to approximately 5,000 steps. By simply choosing to park further from the entrance, I could effortlessly increase my daily step count. This minor adjustment to my daily routine demonstrated that incorporating more activity into my day did not require significant changes, just a more mindful approach to the opportunities for movement already present in my regular schedule.

Turning it into a game, I began to experiment: How far did I need to park to ensure I met my daily step goal? This playful strategy not only helped me consistently surpass the 10,000-step mark but also transformed my approach to physical activity. By intentionally parking further from the entrance, the extra steps accumulated quickly. Through a year of consistent effort, this simple yet effective tactic contributed to a significant milestone—I lost 35 pounds. It took another ten years to find a wellness specialist who helped me understand the role of nutrition and eating. Before long, I finally got back to my 30-year-old weight.

The journey didn't stop there. It took another decade to cross paths with a wellness specialist who illuminated the crucial interplay between nutrition and dietary habits. With his guidance, I delved deeper into understanding how what I ate impacted my health and well-being. This newfound knowledge, combined with my established habit of staying active, eventually led me back to the weight I was in my 30s. The process was gradual, requiring patience and persistence, but it underscored a valuable lesson: achieving and maintaining a healthy weight is a multifaceted endeavor that balances physical activity with mindful nutrition.

I now maintain 135 pounds rather than the 185 pounds I was when I first decided *enough is enough.* I felt sluggish all the time at 185 pounds. Feeling that way makes it difficult to find the motivation to make changes. Sheer determination that this was not my life had been the guiding force, along with finally asking, *If not now, when*? And answering *NOW!*

The reality is you just need to do something. It doesn't matter where you are today. It matters what you want in your future.

If you want perfect health and don't have it today, then start your research immediately. What are you doing right now that is not compatible with your desire for perfect health?

I can already hear the questions pouring in: 'Have you seen the price of healthy food choices? I can't afford that.' 'I can't just leave the house and go to the gym looking like this.' And there are many other questions that naturally arise on this topic.

The key is to start small. Choose one manageable change and begin today. If it involves breaking an existing habit, aim to reduce it gradually.

One vivid example from my life is my excessive caffeine consumption. At one point, I found myself consuming more than seventeen cups of coffee daily. The high-stress nature of my job, where I felt a constant need for caffeine's energizing boost to remain alert and effective, fueled this habit.

One day, I confronted the reality that my caffeine consumption might be detrimental to my health. Around that time, numerous articles emerged, discussing the adverse effects of excessive caffeine intake. According to these articles, the recommended healthy limit was four to five cups a day—a threshold I significantly exceeded.

I switched to water. I went cold turkey. And for one week, I was miserable. I had something similar to delirium tremens (DTs) experienced when you're an alcoholic going through withdrawal. Headaches and flu-like symptoms as well. It was a drag. But at the end of the week, I no longer needed the caffeine.

In response, I made the drastic switch to water, opting to quit caffeine cold turkey. The subsequent week proved to be an ordeal. My withdrawal symptoms mirrored those of delirium tremens (DTs), typically associated with alcohol withdrawal, including severe headaches and flu-like symptoms. This period was incredibly challenging, to say the least.

However, as difficult as that week was, it marked a turning point. By its conclusion, I discovered that my dependency on caffeine had vanished. What started as a grueling test of willpower ended with a liberating freedom from caffeine, showcasing the resilience of the human body and the power of making a health-conscious decision.

I don't recommend following that example, as this was a horrible way to get off anything. It is a tremendous strain on your body. And for those with hidden medical conditions, it could even trigger a catastrophic failure of your nervous system. So my recommendation is to instead remove things gradually. That is also true for adding things to your daily routine.

A more practical approach unfolded like this: If, for example, I consumed seventeen cups of coffee yesterday, today's goal would be to reduce that number to fifteen or sixteen cups, maintaining this new level for a few days. Then after a few days, cut down again to thirteen or fourteen cups of coffee, and continue this pattern of gradual reduction.

This method of incremental decrease allows the body ample time to adapt to each new level of caffeine consumption without shock. By slowly lowering the amount of coffee each day, you minimize the risk of experiencing severe withdrawal symptoms. This gradual adjustment process not only makes the transition more manageable but also significantly increases the likelihood of adhering to the plan.

Affordable nutritious food can often be found through a bit of research. Many areas host farmer's markets offering locally grown produce at lower prices than supermarkets. Additionally, some local farmers allow you to "pick your own" fruits and vegetables, offering a discount for your efforts. This approach not only supports local agriculture but also makes incorporating fresh, healthy food into your diet more budget-friendly.

Watch for special deals at your local grocery store. Many grocery stores offer special days for senior citizens that include discounts on different products. If you are a senior, take advantage of that option to help you save money. Be sure to stock up on anything with a long shelf life, such as canned, boxed, or frozen foods. You may need to do some research and find what options are available to you. Don't fret over the small things. There are ways to move to a better quality of food without breaking the bank. It is a matter of researching and staying cognizant of what is available in your area.

In a rural area, you may have more choices than in an urban area. Just make the changes you can and see the impact.

Next, when starting an exercise program, you may find the camaraderie and structure of a gym helps to keep you on track. However, a gym membership is not a requirement to get healthy. Remember the 10K challenge I mentioned? That was 10,000 steps per day. You could do it walking or running. I dropped most of the weight, doing nothing more than walking 10,000 steps daily.

No time or money for the gym? There are lots of videos to choose from. YouTube channels and programs on TV offer opportunities for you to get fit and stay fit from the comfort of your own home.

If you are someone who hasn't exercised in a long time, please see your doctor before starting any exercise program. Your doctor can also advise you on programs and exercises that can help your condition along with ones you should avoid. Physical health and well-being can get you where you want to go much quicker than other things you have tried in the past.

Weights for your home exercise routines can be created with household items like a twenty-ounce bottle of water. That's a little over a pound you can use as a hand weight. A gallon of water or milk is approximately eight pounds. I think you get the idea that it is possible to keep costs down and still get in the exercise you need with a little ingenuity. Refill empty bottles with sand and water to make them even heavier. So your homemade exercise equipment can grow with you (up to a point).

Exercise encompasses any activity that involves muscle movement, extending beyond weight training to include walking or gentle stretching. Such activities not only promote fitness but also help in staying pain-free by massaging and moving different muscle groups.

Gentle stretching allows lactic acid to move out of the muscles where it can build up if you do any strenuous exercise. In my experience, strenuous exercise is not a requirement for good health. Moving every day is the key factor.

What does that mean? Consider hip circles, arm circles, neck circles. These simple exercises move your hips, arms, and neck and keep the fluid inside flowing and the muscles limber. I would suggest starting with ten of each exercise once or twice a day. Be sure to go in both directions, left and right, on the hip and neck circles. Forward, then backward, on the arm circles. It won't take a long time yet it can have significant health benefits in the long run.

Toe-touching exercises can be performed either standing up and reaching towards the floor or sitting down and bending over your legs to touch your toes. To do this, bend toward your toes for a count of five, then straighten back up for another count of five. Aim to gradually increase your endurance until you can maintain the bend for a count of thirty. Repeat this process ten times, once or twice daily. These exercises should be executed slowly and deliberately, without any bouncing movements. Bouncing is not recommended as it can easily cause tears or sprains. While younger individuals may recover quickly from such injuries, for those in their fifties or older, the same injuries could result in long-term pain.

Regardless of age, adopting a gentle and slow approach to all exercises is advisable. High-impact exercises, which often involve jumping and can exert undue stress on the lower body, particularly the knees, are not recommended. There are numerous alternative strategies to intensify a workout without resorting to high-impact movements. These methods include wearing a weight vest to add resistance, using hand weights during exercises to increase difficulty, and holding positions for extended periods, over 30 seconds, to enhance strength and endurance.

Keep in mind, younger individuals tend to recover from injuries much faster than older adults. The goal of exercising is to enhance your health while keeping your life pain-free. To achieve this, it's crucial to steer clear of activities that are deemed dangerous, pose a risk of injury, or force your body into unnatural positions.

If you ever find yourself questioning whether you're performing an exercise correctly, consulting a professional is a wise step. Consider scheduling a session with a personal trainer. You can also visit your local gym and seek recommendations from the professionals there. Their expertise can guide you toward safe and effective exercise techniques, ensuring that you achieve your health goals without compromising your well-being.

When you notice that your current exercise routine no longer challenges you as it once did, it's not an indication that the routine is ineffective. Rather, it suggests that your muscles have adapted to the regimen, diminishing its impact. This is a natural part of the exercise process and signals it's time to introduce new exercises to shake things up. By swapping out familiar exercises for new ones, you target different, yet complementary, muscle groups, reinvigorating your workout and ensuring continued progress.

The goal is to maintain pain-free mobility for life. While certain physical conditions may limit some activities, most people can benefit significantly from a consistent, simple exercise plan. Such a plan not only promises a life with less pain but also enhances overall enjoyment of life, underscoring the importance of staying active and adaptable in your fitness journey.

For example, those in a wheelchair, who are not quadriplegic, can do arm circles, toe touches, neck circles, etc. Over time, they can add upper-body strength-training exercises as well. Those not steady on their feet can do a lot of their exercises while sitting down. They can also add lower-body exercises such as flutter kicks from a seated position. An exercise therapist can offer other options for adjusting exercises for a specific physical impairment.

So what's your plan for living a long and pain-free life? Are you going to start today? You don't need to make it difficult.

What can you commit to? Are you all in, or do you need to keep thinking about this? Hoping and praying that something will change without realizing that you picked up this book as an inspiration. What are you waiting for?

What is stopping you? Maybe it's fear. Fear of the unknown or fear that if you change your health for the better, you'll lose friends, or that you won't be you anymore.

What I am saying is that you need to examine your situation and figure out why you are so resistant to moving forward with improving your health. Is it because being sick and tired gives you the perfect excuse not to do certain things? Because it keeps you from having to take part in certain activities.

Maybe it just seems easier than having to actually say, 'I don't want to do that.' If people see you getting healthy while everyone around you is following unhealthy practices, you might feel peer pressure to go back to your old ways of being.

Believe me, the universe does not want you sick and tired.

For example, maybe your challenge is a venti Starbucks mocha latte at 530 calories when made with whole milk, or a large piece of cheesecake (510 calories). These are two of my favorites and helped me add fifty pounds to my small frame.

I don't want you to think you can't have your favorite treat. What I am saying is that you can't have your favorite treat every day. In my case, I will have that piece of cheesecake once a month. The Starbucks coffee I gave up, along with my seventeen-cup-a-day coffee habit. I have since found fresh fruit makes a much more satisfying treat than either the coffee or the cheesecake. And a much healthier option as well.

Fill in the blank for your weakness. You know what's causing you to say, "No thanks. I'm going to stay where I am. I don't want to move on. I can't move on. You just don't understand my situation."

That is likely true. I can't fully understand your situation because I'm not you, but just because I didn't live through that disease, that trauma, that pain you are experiencing, doesn't mean what I'm saying is any less relevant to your situation. It is up to you to stop looking for excuses and decide right now. What do you really want out of this life?

You get one life of unknown length, and it's up to you to use your time wisely. If fitness and health are not a priority for you, then continue down the path you're on. However, if you decide enough is enough and you are sick and tired of being sick and tired, then consider making some tweaks to your current routine.

If you want to improve your chances of a disease-free life, or a life without debilitating illness, consider starting a personal nutrition and exercise program. Research shows that many common diseases, such as diabetes, heart disease, and the like, result from poor nutrition and exercise choices. These choices ultimately wear down the organs and cause them to fail.

I want to be healthy in my nineties and beyond, and if you have read this far, I believe you do too.

Take that first step today. Your body will appreciate it and, over time, so will you.

Now that we've addressed the objections, what else is holding you back? You can start at home using what's available. Taking walks can be both fun and a way to meet the neighbors. If you're walking around your neighborhood, you'll start feeling better in no time at all.

As you begin to feel better, your attitude will improve, providing you with more energy and a renewed sense of confidence to advance to the next stage of your life. When you were feeling sick and tired all the time, you had less energy and interest in trying new activities.

Yes, certain conditions, like tinnitus and vertigo, may not change, but other issues, particularly those related to excess weight or inactivity, will gradually improve. As you start feeling more like your former self, people around you will take notice. Some may even ask, "Have you done something different? What is it? I know! It's a new blouse, or maybe a haircut?"

I can't make you take action. My role is to help you understand what's at stake and offer suggestions on how to begin and what activities to pursue. I can even open the door for you. However, it's up to you to step through that door and declare, "I am here! I am ready! I am doing this for my health." Only then will real change occur.

Chapter Exercise:

Take fifteen minutes to journal about these questions. Focus on what you want to look like and feel like as you age.

What would you do if you found yourself with a debilitating health challenge and couldn't get any answers from the professionals?

Would you stand up and say "I can take anything you can dish out" to the universe?

Work on finding your own answers to give meaning to your life.

Chapter Five

The rest of the story

When I was a child, my podiatrist warned me that surgery might eventually become necessary. By 2017, the RICE method (rest, ice, compression, elevation) was no longer effective; my instep remained in a constant state of 'sprain,' causing persistent pain with each step. After thorough research, I consulted with a podiatrist who concurred that surgery to remove the extra bones was the best course of action. The procedure went smoothly, as planned.

The cast was removed eight weeks post-surgery, initiating a four-week period of gradually increasing weight on my foot. This phase was succeeded by four months of physical therapy to restore full functionality. A cane was instrumental in helping me maintain balance and ensure proper foot alignment throughout this recovery phase.

In April 2018, I had the opportunity to attend an International Living conference in Atlanta, Georgia. The conference was an enlightening experience, offering insights into living abroad and connecting attendees with individuals who had embarked on such adventures. It was inspiring to meet both singles and couples who had ventured beyond the United States and Canada in search of adventure and had no intentions of returning.

It was an incredible three days, and though I was walking with a cane, it was not preventing me from doing anything.

I was excited about the prospect that at the next doctor's appointment, the doctor would say I could stop using the cane. I felt invincible and believed I would soon return to my old self, which meant fast walking, one-hour gym workouts, and resuming all the other activities I had put on hold while recuperating from foot surgery.

I never saw the dark shadow appearing on the horizon. It was a typical sunny day in Florida, but I was in unbearable pain. A deafening noise plagued my left ear, and an intense pain pulsed through my head. Despite feeling fine the day before, I was suddenly overwhelmed with symptoms reminiscent of the flu, hoping it would soon pass. I initially dismissed the idea of seeking immediate medical attention.

However, as my condition worsened over two weeks, marked by nausea, vomiting, and dizziness, I recognized the need to consult a doctor. Unfortunately, it was the weekend, and my doctor's office was closed, but the walk-in clinic was available.

Upon reviewing my symptoms, the clinic staff urged me to visit the ER, fearing a potentially serious condition like meningitis. They were concerned that treating what appeared to be an ear infection with antibiotics might be dangerously insufficient, risking severe consequences.

Though I understood the clinic's need for caution, I was annoyed at having to go to the ER and endure another wait to see a doctor. I took their note and headed straight to the ER, where I signed in. Upon reviewing my symptoms, the staff decided I needed blood work. Fifteen minutes later,

I had my blood drawn and blood pressure checked. They then found a room in the back for my husband and me to wait, during which time I felt increasingly worse. Finally, the doctor arrived and began asking questions.

"Have you been out of the country? Been around any exotic animals?" among other questions that seemed irrelevant to me. No, I hadn't traveled abroad recently, though I had attended a conference six weeks prior with many international attendees. No, I hadn't visited the zoo or been knowingly exposed to anyone sick. My mind raced with thoughts of the rare and exotic diseases I could have encountered at the conference.

After completing his checklist, the doctor examined my left ear and exclaimed, "Lady, you have a lake going on back there," before prescribing antibiotics for an ear infection and sending me on my way. In some respects, I felt relieved. It was "just" an ear infection, nothing as severe as meningitis. I understood now; the clinic's caution was driven by the fear of legal repercussions should their diagnosis be incorrect.

One week after completing the antibiotics, with no improvement in my condition, I scheduled an appointment with my primary care physician. He reviewed my medical history and recommended seeing an ear specialist. I managed to secure an appointment for the following week, the earliest available.

On the day of the appointment, a technician first assessed my situation and suggested that the sequence of tests I was about to undergo was incorrect; a hearing test should have been conducted initially to detect any hearing impairments. Following this advice, I underwent a hearing test, which revealed hearing impairments.

While the discovery of hearing loss was valuable, my primary concern was addressing the persistent noise in my left ear and the accompanying vertigo. The doctor explained that both symptoms were due to a disparity in hearing between my two ears. Specifically, there was a loss of hearing in the lower frequencies of my left ear. As a result, my left ear was generating noise to compensate for the missing sounds, in an attempt to align with what the right ear was hearing.

This misalignment was causing my body significant difficulty in trying to synchronize these divergent auditory inputs, leading to the vertigo. The challenge lay in the body's struggle to reconcile these two different perceptions of the auditory world.

I also mentioned that I was having trouble sleeping because the tinnitus (noise in my left ear) was so loud it kept me awake. The doctor didn't have answers for me. Instead, he decided to set me up for more tests.

In the meantime, I turned to meditation, hoping it might alleviate any stress that could be worsening my condition. The thought of the extreme consequences of prolonged sleep deprivation—hallucinations and, in rare cases, death—was alarming.

My meditation routine was straightforward: I would lie on the bed, eyes closed, with the sound of a soothing babbling brook playing in the background. After a couple of weeks of consistent meditation, I began to notice an improvement. Gradually, I was able to sleep for longer stretches at a time, despite the relentless noise that resembled a helicopter buzzing next to my ear. Initially, I managed only four hours of sleep a night, but after six months, I was able to return to my usual seven hours most nights.

While I found some relief through meditation, my doctor was diligently working to determine the next steps. Typically, ear infections do not lead to hearing loss, prompting them to order a comprehensive series of tests. After undergoing numerous examinations that left me feeling poked, prodded, and exhausted, I was still without answers for my persistent ear pain and the irritating ringing. The doctor decided to proceed with more diagnostic tests, including an MRI, in search of a solution.

The answer to those tests was the same: Everything looked normal. They could not find anything wrong with me.

However, I still experienced ringing in my ear and vertigo, which made me nauseous and gave me the sensation of falling.

Then, after numerous tests, the ear doctor dismissed me via an encrypted message on the patient portal. Can you imagine that? Coming home to find a message instructing you to visit your doctor's portal for more information.

The message stated he had exhausted all potential treatments. It acknowledged hearing loss of unknown origin, with a caveat that I was over fifty years old. He concluded that since all the tests indicated everything appeared normal, there was nothing more he could do for me. There was no point in scheduling any more appointments.

Think about it. You're desperately looking for answers.

Wondering why me?

What happened?

Why did this happen?

How did this happen?

Could I have done something differently?

Could this happen to the other ear?

Will I become fully deaf?

How do I solve this?

The response I received from the expert felt dismissive, as if he were saying, "Sorry, kid, go away, you're bothering me." To make matters worse, the doctor seemed to imply that being over fifty was in itself a diagnosis.

Fortunately, around that time, a coworker mentioned the specialist her husband was seeing for a similarly mysterious ear issue, who was actually providing help. Seizing this ray of hope, I immediately made an appointment with this new ear specialist. I brought along some of my medical records to the first appointment, where he conducted another hearing test since it had been four months since my last one. However, he found no change in my condition.

He explained that the disparity in hearing between my left and right ears was responsible for my feeling of imbalance. Curious, he inquired why I was using a cane, wondering if I also had a lower body issue. I clarified that the cane was initially for support following foot surgery a year prior. Due to my difficulty discerning whether I was standing upright or falling over in open spaces, I had resumed using the cane as a precautionary measure. Essentially, it was the difference between the stability of a ladder and the uncertainty of a three-legged stool.

The ladder needs to lean against something, like a building, to be useful, whereas the three-legged stool stands independently. Given that I only have two legs, I recognized the necessity of a third point of contact with the ground to confirm my upright stance. The cane offered the added advantage of helping maintain my cognitive focus.Before consistently using the cane outdoors, taking a step would trigger a barrage of internal questions: "OK, arms, are we still upright? Legs, are we still upright?" and so on, involving the entire body. This process was not only time-consuming but also physically draining. Unless I was seated in a stable and safe setting, my mind would incessantly repeat these questions, potentially hundreds or even thousands of times a day.

Consequently, there was little mental capacity left for other considerations, such as work, my side project of writing a book, deciding what to have for dinner, or any other aspect of daily life. Everything else was overshadowed by the constant concern: Am I upright, or am I falling? This situation was untenable, and I realized the need for a solution.

The doctor wanted me to take drugs.

I explained to him that I had issues with medications. In fact, I would prefer to avoid taking drugs altogether. Medications have had severely negative impacts on my body, just shy of being fatal. Depending on the medication, I would either experience the most severe side effect, short of death, or the complete opposite of the expected side effect.

For instance, he prescribed a diuretic, and after only four days, I nearly passed out and struggled to get out of bed because it had removed not just the water but all the salt from my system. Clearly, this was not a viable solution for me. In this instance, the drug was too effective at removing water, which was the problem rather than the potential side effects.

When I next visited the doctor, he suggested trying a medication typically used for epilepsy. He said, "This drug has drowsiness as a side effect and is going to work great for you!" At that desperate point, I almost refused. However, he assured me that the dosage he prescribed was the lowest possible and that it was a solid pill, which I could cut in half if I wanted to start with a smaller dose. I filled the prescription that afternoon.

It was Friday when my doctor recommended taking the pill just before bed, assuring me it would induce sleep within fifteen minutes. Heeding his advice, I took half a pill and attempted to settle in for the night. Contrary to expectations, sleep eluded me, leaving me feeling as though I'd been electrified by a thousand bolts of lightning. Restlessness took over, and after an unsuccessful hour of trying to sleep, I abandoned the effort and turned to house cleaning. Remarkably, in just three hours, I had rendered my entire house immaculate.

At this point, my husband urged me to try and rest, concerned by the fact I had been awake for at least eighteen hours, which was out of character for me. Fortunately, it was now Saturday, so there was no work obligation. Despite lying back in bed with him, my mind continued to race, making it impossible for me to relax. Eventually, he fell asleep, and I returned to my home office to work on my budget. I managed to review my finances and pay all my bills, then shifted my focus to developing a business plan and imagining its potential.

As dawn approached, I began researching the side effects of the medication I had taken, convinced that something in it must have triggered this overwhelming sense of euphoria and mania.

Instead, I found the side effects to be exactly as the doctor had initially warned. The label cautioned, "This can cause drowsiness. Do not take it if planning on operating heavy machinery." However, in my case, the side effect was the exact opposite of drowsiness.

This state of heightened alertness persisted for hours, astonishingly keeping me wide awake. Finally, around 3:00 PM on Saturday afternoon, I crashed. Literally. My husband discovered me lying on the floor in my office.

By then, I had been awake for thirty-three consecutive hours. My husband, believing he was helping, insisted I move to the couch. That's when the situation deteriorated dramatically. I was hit with an immediate and excruciating migraine, which brought on nausea and vomiting.

I found myself on the bathroom floor, clinging to the toilet for the next hour. Having not eaten for at least eighteen hours, I experienced nothing but dry heaves, exacerbating my misery. Lying on the cold bathroom tiles, the chill penetrated my legs and hips. Each time I attempted to find a comfortable position, I was overcome by the urge to vomit again. My emotions oscillated between laughter and tears—laughter at the absurdity of one half of a tiny pill causing such havoc, and tears from the excruciating pain I was enduring.

I finally felt stable enough to leave the bathroom and crawled on my hands and knees to the couch. Once there, I asked my husband to bring me a cold cloth for my forehead, which I also used to shield my eyes from the light. What a mess. I had never felt so terrible in my life. The worst case of whiplash I had experienced was nothing compared to this agony, even with its accompanying neck and back spasms that had previously brought me to tears.

I lay on the couch, enduring what felt like an eternity, waiting for both the couch and the room to stop spinning. Of course, neither was actually moving, but my senses were so skewed that I even confirmed this with my husband.

Finally, the spinning ceased. I chose to remain still for another hour before my hunger became overwhelming.

But it was more than hunger; I was "hangry." Still, wanting to avoid taxing my body further, I opted for a bowl of rice with a small amount of butter, considering it bland enough and the fat necessary for my body's needs. I went to bed immediately afterward and fell asleep as soon as my head hit the pillow, sleeping for eighteen hours. I awoke for a few hours on Sunday, ate a small meal, and then returned to bed, hoping to be well enough to work on Monday. By Monday, I wasn't fully recovered, but I decided to go to work anyway.

Barely functioning

My day job didn't notice I was barely functioning, which was fortunate. Or perhaps I am such an overachiever that on a day when I was merely okay, my office considered my output acceptable, even though I wasn't meeting my personal standards. After returning home that night, I had a small meal and then slept for ten hours. On Tuesday morning, feeling slightly better than I had all week, one of the first things I did was send a message to the doctor informing him that I had stopped taking the pill. I mentioned the side effects and stated that we could discuss other options during my appointment on Friday.

On Friday, the doctor was puzzled by my experience. After I recounted the entire ordeal, he mentioned he had spoken with a colleague at Johns Hopkins, who suggested that since I was prone to migraines, I should try a migraine diet. By this point, I was quite skeptical about finding a resolution to my symptoms.

I agreed that a change in diet was doable and certainly preferable to further risky encounters with medication. He handed me a two-page document containing a few links and general information but no specific details on what a migraine diet entails or how to implement it..

After paying these professionals for assistance, this was the best they could offer? So much for care and compassion in the healthcare industry. I took the document home, hoping perhaps one link would lead to a website detailing the diet. Unfortunately, the links merely directed me to a clinic at Johns Hopkins in Baltimore, MD. Living in Florida, this was not particularly helpful.

The links provided were to medical journal articles detailing patient experiences with the migraine diet and their outcomes. While these stories were intriguing, they lacked specific details about the diet itself—what foods to include or avoid. This lack of information led me to conduct my own research via "Doctor Google," a testament to why many people hesitate to consult medical professionals until absolutely necessary.

Through my research, I discovered several resources outlining the migraine diet and its principles. I purchased a couple of well-reviewed books on Amazon to delve deeper. Remarkably, by identifying potential migraine triggers and focusing on benign foods, I experienced a significant turnaround in my condition.

The migraine diet was a key part of the solution. I eliminated several foods, many of which I seldom ate. However, cutting out favorites like raspberries, identified as potential triggers, was challenging. Fortunately, the diet still allowed for a wide variety of other fruits and vegetables. The migraine diet closely resembles the Mediterranean diet, enabling me to maintain healthy eating habits.

In essence, both the Mediterranean and Migraine diets emphasize fruits, vegetables, and healthy fats like olive and coconut oil. Proteins primarily come from fish, though no meat is strictly prohibited. I also chose to reduce my salt intake to lower water retention risks, keeping my daily sodium consumption around 1200 mg.

Despite the persistent ringing in my ears, the sleeplessness and migraines that had been constant companions began to subside. Gradually, I found a sense of normalcy, or at least a new normal, which included using a cane in public. Not due to any issues with my lower body, but because it helped my brain relax, eliminating the need to constantly check if I was maintaining balance. This significant change afforded me the confidence to venture out in public without fear.

The improvement was remarkable. I could now step outside, go to work, visit stores, or travel anywhere I desired without worry. However, after some time, the progress reached a plateau. While I wasn't fully recovered, I felt significantly better than I had since the ordeal began in 2018.

Chapter Exercise:

Take thirty minutes for this journaling exercise.

Review your eating patterns. Are you eating a balanced diet, or whatever is easy?

Are you ready to make some changes and add exercise to your daily routine?

What can you do today that will improve your situation?

Make a list.

Chapter Six
And then...

So, what's next? The concepts of a perfect day and perfect health are intertwined. This leads us to a crucial inquiry: How can one enjoy a perfect day without good health?

To me, perfect health is reminiscent of the days before my left ear suffered hearing loss, before the onset of tinnitus, and before the vertigo battles began. It was a time when I could step outside without the need to clutch a cane for fear that, in an open space, my brain would incessantly query each part of my body, "Are we falling?"

Initially, a mere 30 minutes outside would leave me drained, and my disdain for venturing out intensified with each experience. However, the cane changed everything. It provided my brain with a third point of contact with the ground, fostering a sense of security.

With the cane, I found peace. I could navigate the outdoors silently, allowing me to shop, work in the office, or park my car without feeling exhausted by the time I reached my destination. My brain was at ease, no longer plagued by the fear of falling. Recent hearing tests have shown slight improvements in my left ear, a positive development that enhances my safety when crossing busy streets. Yet, vertigo remains a daily challenge, one I must continuously manage.

Perfect health

Let's take a moment to reflect on what we truly desire from life. Do you wish to persist in a state of stress, constantly anxious about your health, gradually withdrawing into isolation?

Do you want to dedicate your life solely to work, toiling away to cover expenses, yet finding no happiness in your daily existence?

What if there was a better way? What if there was an easy button that changed everything?

Envision perfect health: a life free from dependency on daily prescription medications, possibly supplemented by just a multivitamin or a couple of nutritional supplements. Understandably, this ideal might not be attainable for everyone.

For those reliant on prescription medications, it's crucial to consult with your medical team before making any changes. Perhaps you're a transplant recipient who requires anti-rejection drugs to protect your new organ, or maybe you're a diabetic dependent on insulin shots to manage your blood sugar levels. There are numerous reasons why individuals must take prescription drugs on a regular basis. However, this doesn't preclude you from exploring other options. Conducting research and discussing with your doctor the possibility of non-prescription alternatives for your condition is advisable. There may be lifestyle or dietary adjustments capable of diminishing your reliance on prescription medications.

Despite your limitations, with proper care, you can achieve good health for your situation.

Next on the list is a regular diet and exercise routine.

When choosing what to eat, I prioritize fresh or frozen organic options to minimize exposure to pesticides and other contaminants, aligning with the core principles of organic farming. This approach emphasizes raising animals and cultivating vegetables without the use of pesticides or antibiotics. Research indicates that pesticides and antibiotics can contribute to a broad spectrum of illnesses. Additionally, the routine administration of antibiotics to animals has been identified as a contributing factor to the emergence of antibiotic-resistant bacteria.

During the growing season, visiting the local farmers' market provides access to fresh produce directly from the field. Consuming higher-quality food not only improves your overall health but also supports the local community by offering fresher options and bolstering local farmers.

I love the outdoors and make it a point to go for a walk daily. This routine serves dual purposes: fulfilling my daily exercise needs and ensuring I get enough vitamin D, which is crucial for preventing rickets, a disease resulting from vitamin D deficiency.

Incorporating gentle, slow stretching before and after the walk enhances overall health benefits, making this exercise regimen not only safe for a broad range of individuals but also effective in boosting stamina and flexibility.

Remember, it's important to undergo a physical examination annually to identify any potential health issues early. Additionally, if your yearly check-up doesn't include it, make sure to schedule a skin cancer screening, especially if you have a family history of cancer or spend significant time outdoors without sunscreen.

For me, a perfect day is spent in a tropical paradise, where the temperature hovers in the pleasant range of the 70s and 80s during the day, allowing me to dress in a skirt and short-sleeve shirt for formal occasions. My everyday wear consists of shorts and a short-sleeve shirt, with a jacket seldom needed aside from a raincoat. And even then, the rain is often warm, tempting me to step out without a coat and deliberately enjoy getting caught in a rainstorm.

This paradise could be in the southern United States or anywhere else in the world with that kind of climate.

Chapter Exercise

Grab your journal and consider the following scenario. Think back to when you were healthy. You got up every morning feeling great. You would jump out of bed, excited to start your day. Compare that to where you are today.

After sitting with this concept for about fifteen minutes, journal your answers.

This exercise gets you out of your head and brings awareness to what you want your life to look like.

Take some time each day and envision living a life where you enjoy your time on this earth.

What is one thing you will do today to ensure you maintain your health for as long as you live?

Chapter Seven
Dream Life

This chapter is a projection of what I would like my life to look like after getting my health challenges under control.

I aspire to wake up every day pain-free, with all my body parts functioning as they did when I was a teenager. I want to take long walks in the woods without worrying about how long it will take to reach the waterfall. I want to dance until midnight without needing to ice my knee or call a doctor the next day due to a sprain or strain. More than anything, I desire the assurance that my body can handle these activities without drama or pain, and that I won't regret attempting them the following day, plagued by suffering.

I long for the simplicity of running errands—to the grocery store, the bank, and the gas station—carrying bags of groceries into the house effortlessly, without pain or complications. I yearn to go on bike rides without the fear of falling. All this is what I want.

I seek the ability to be active and enjoy life, unhampered by health challenges or the fear of what might happen.

What follows is my hypothetical perfect day.

My ideal day unfolds on the veranda, with a breathtaking view of a pristine white sandy beach where the ocean waves gently caress the shore. I enjoy a breakfast of fresh fruit and cottage cheese, basking in the serenity. A soft ocean breeze wafts by, and birds soar joyfully in the sky. I am enveloped in peace.

An hour later, after breakfast, I head inside to prepare for a client meeting. I assist the client in overcoming their mindset blocks concerning money and financial freedom, and together, we develop a plan for their continued progress post-session.

Since its inception a decade ago, my business has experienced significant growth. I've expanded the team and even begun franchising internationally. Despite this expansion, I ensure the integrity of our course material, requiring all franchisees to use the same platform for ease of adding new programs and maintaining software consistency. Franchisees have the autonomy to set their course prices, but I've established a minimum charge to preserve the value of our signature program and maintain fairness across the franchise network.

I finish organizing my tasks for the day and decide to take a stroll around my property. I own a two-acre plot of land with a three-bedroom, two-bathroom house situated on a hill overlooking the ocean. Each morning, I wake up to the sight of beautiful birds and fresh fruit on the trees. The temperature hovers in the mid-70s during the day and mid-60s at night.

I can wear shorts and a light top every day, fully embracing the Southern hospitality. My home is close enough to town that I often walk there to see what's new at the market. Frequently, I'll pick up something for dinner that night instead of buying a week's worth of groceries in advance.

My new lifestyle affords me the opportunity to exercise and obtain fresh food for my daily meals simultaneously. It represents a significant departure from my previous way of life.

My diet is carefully chosen to maintain my health, incorporating elements of both the Mediterranean and Migraine diets.

Olive oil and coconut oil, as 'good fats,' have become my allies. I've discovered that consuming foods not recommended by either the Mediterranean or Migraine diets causes me distress. Items labeled as "avoid" on the migraine diet, especially when consumed in large quantities or too frequently, will trigger migraines. Thus, I steer clear of these triggers, allowing me to feel well and enjoy my life.

What would your dream life look like if you just opened your mind to the possibilities that everything is available to you?

Envision your life if financial constraints were nonexistent. What activities would you pursue if your family and friends supported your decisions?

Whatever it might be, could you commit 100 percent to this new idea, this new way of living?

Or are you so deeply ingrained in a mindset of scarcity and deficiency that you cannot envision a different future for yourself? How can there be any improvement? It's disheartening to think that fear might prevent you from sharing your unique gifts with the world.

Reflect deeply on what is preventing you from embracing change. What holds you back from living the life you dream of? Are external factors such as friends or family influencing you, or is it an internal struggle? Perhaps you've attempted something similar in the past that didn't pan out. Or maybe, someone in your family took a risk and is now ostracized, becoming the cautionary tale of what not to pursue in life.

What is *really* stopping you?

You must confront and acknowledge your fear to overcome it. If you don't, you'll remain stagnant, and so will those who could benefit from your help.

Don't allow fear to keep you hidden. Step out from the shadows, confront your fears, and boldly move toward your goals. Achieving them is not an unattainable fantasy; it's a genuine possibility that lies within you.

You have something unique that needs to be shared with the world. This message could inspire and impact thousands, if not millions. Yet, you're concealing your potential due to fear: fear of the unknown, fear of failure, fear of losing friends, or fear that your ideas won't be accepted.

Why let fear dictate your actions?

The impact of fear on our lives can tie us up in knots, yet overcoming it begins with a single step, much like the ascent of a mountain. So, what's your first step? Is it conducting research on your target market, or identifying your ideal customer? Consider what truly ignites your passion. What is it that makes your heart sing?

What makes you want to get out of bed in the morning?

If you could spend your day doing what you love, it would feel more like play than work, enriching your life immeasurably. I recall a seminar where this concept was discussed, and the idea resonated deeply with me: the notion of being so engrossed in your work that it ceases to feel like labor.

Indeed, work is essential for generating income to cover expenses, but it's crucial to find joy in your professional endeavors. This balance is key to maintaining an efficient and effective business, ensuring employee satisfaction if you choose to expand your team. But have you envisioned what your business would look like?

What steps will lead you to financial independence? While many people have a vision for their ideal life, few take the necessary actions to achieve it. Instead of actively pursuing their dreams, they rely on wishful thinking, hoping for fortune to magically appear. They might even resort to buying lottery tickets or engaging in other games of chance, never explicitly stating their desires or considering the power of writing them down.

What about creating a plan to realize your goals? Where do you stand with your financial planning? Have you taken the time to write it down, to clarify whether you see your future as an employee or as an entrepreneur? Do you have a clear vision of what you aspire to be?

Some of you might have crafted vision boards, while others have written affirmations to place on your bathroom mirror. Despite these efforts, you might find that nothing significant has changed. Perhaps you've watched *The Secret*, read numerous books on the law of attraction, and yet, it all seems ineffective, leading you to dismiss these ideas as impractical marketing fluff without any real-world application.

But what if the key component you're missing is your *mindset?*

Your starting point, where you currently find yourself, and what you truly believe in can dramatically influence the success of your financial planning. Your mindset is the foundation upon which all your financial decisions and plans are built.

Chapter Exercise:

Grab your journal and set aside fifteen minutes for this exercise. Visualize this scenario then journal about it.

What would a perfect day look like for you? A day in which your medical condition is under control, you are doing what you love, whether you are working or enjoying leisure time.

Chapter Eight
Yet more tests

Sometimes, you might feel stuck with your medical team, undergoing numerous tests only for each to return inconclusive or to indicate that nothing is wrong. Everything appears normal, leaving you without a diagnosis.

You're aware something isn't right. Why else would you experience pain? It could be a persistent ringing in your ear, vertigo, or other less visible issues that, because they can't be seen, aren't treated as legitimate concerns. Worse yet, you might be told it's all in your head.

You may hear statements like, "We can't find anything wrong, so we'll prescribe these anxiety pills, as you seem overly anxious about this."

The experience of feeling dismissed by your doctor varies from person to person. Do you start to doubt yourself when the doctor says the tests show nothing wrong? Their response doesn't alter the reality that you're facing a significant, life-altering challenge.

Remember, it's your body and your quality of life.

You have the right to seek second opinions, third opinions, or as many as necessary until you feel all your concerns have been addressed and you can come to terms with your situation.

Navigating medical plans for standard Western medicine can become prohibitively expensive, especially when dealing with an undiagnosed illness. Moreover, finding a doctor who takes your concerns seriously can prove challenging. At times, exploring alternatives outside the Western medical sphere, such as chiropractic care, acupuncture, or other Asian health practices, might provide the solution you're seeking.

Your issue might stem from something as specific as spinal misalignment or even dental problems. It's possible that a misaligned jaw is at the root of your headaches and other symptoms.

The insistence by one medical sector that nothing is amiss doesn't mean you're relegated to enduring your pain indefinitely. The notion of just "sucking it up" need not become your new reality.

Consider how you feel when told, "This is as good as it gets. We've done all we can for now." If you're facing a current dead end, it might merely mean there's a breakthrough just beyond the horizon, yet to be discovered.

If your internal response screams, "There must be an answer," then it's clear your search should continue. If, however, you find yourself thinking, "There are no answers at the moment," perhaps setting a reminder for three months down the line to revisit your research could be beneficial. This journey is uniquely yours, and I cannot dictate which path is best for you. My role is merely to present you with the available options.

The purpose is to allow your body the opportunity to align with your mind and the research you've conducted thus far.

Sometimes, stepping back from the relentless search can lead the answer to reveal itself. It's in those moments of pause, perhaps as brief as the space between raindrops, that solutions can emerge.

At times, the difficult truth may be that there is no definitive answer or cure. The condition you're dealing with might represent the best possible scenario given current medical understanding.

However, the solution could also manifest as a change in diet, an adjustment to your exercise routine, or a comprehensive lifestyle overhaul, revealing itself precisely when it's meant to.

Sometimes, when you struggle, it's natural to seek immediate answers, yet they don't always come right away.

Consider my own experience: I'm still searching for why an ear infection evolved into hearing loss, subsequently causing tinnitus and vertigo, and undermining my independence and self-assurance. I've come to terms with my limitations and have even learned to sleep through the perpetual noise akin to a helicopter in my head, occasionally managing to momentarily forget the tinnitus.

Through gradual steps, I've been rediscovering confidence in myself and my body via vestibular rehabilitation therapy, which aims to recalibrate the brain's perception of movement, thereby reducing vertigo episodes. This therapy was suggested by a neighbor I met during one of my daily walks. Upon mentioning it to my doctor, who then reviewed my medical history, she expressed surprise that this option hadn't been presented to me earlier.

Adapting to life with a health issue is challenging, and initially, it's difficult to find any positive aspect in experiencing hearing loss in one ear, tinnitus, and vertigo. However, after years of contemplation, I've identified a silver lining in this ordeal.

The vertigo has compelled me to slow down and truly appreciate life and the blessings I have: the possessions I cherish, and the people in my life who support me unconditionally. These are individuals who do not judge me for using a cane or assume my capabilities are limited due to migraines, tinnitus, or vertigo. They understand my pace has slowed, and for some, this change has been welcome; previously, my long legs allowed me to stride through walks effortlessly.

For those who have received a diagnosis, various emotions may surface. Fear, perhaps wishing the condition were different. Frustration, anger, or resentment toward the world, or even blaming others for choices that were ultimately your own. What feelings arise for you?

You might feel angry, especially if conditions like diabetes are hereditary in your family, and you realize too late that research and simple lifestyle changes from an early age could have potentially prevented such a diagnosis.

For some, a cancer diagnosis triggers shock and panic, emotions I deeply understand. The overwhelming fear can cloud your ability to process the reality, tempting you to ignore it. Yet, acknowledging the possibility and conducting your own research are crucial steps towards managing the situation. And there's always the slight chance that the initial diagnosis was incorrect, making a second or even third opinion invaluable given the complexity of diseases.

Maybe you need time to sit with the diagnosis.

I recall the first time I faced a cancer scare; I was overwhelmed with terror, finding myself inconsolable and emotionally numb. When the doctor suggested scheduling a biopsy and cryosurgery, I could hardly grasp what was being said, yet I noted the information and ended the call.

Two hours later, the note by the phone reminded me of the hospital appointment scheduled for the following day after work. Despite barely recalling the conversation, I resolved to proceed with the appointment, having already agreed to it.

Following the procedure, the medical team expressed optimism that they had eradicated the issue but recommended a follow-up in one week to discuss the biopsy results. To my immense relief, the biopsy came back negative.

No cancer.

One week later, the second scan at my follow-up appointment confirmed the absence of any additional abnormal cells. I breathed a deep sigh of relief.

How you might navigate a similar situation could vary, but that was how I managed mine: with fright, feeling as if time had frozen, struggling to breathe, overwhelmed by terror. I was convinced my life was at its end. Then came the biopsy, followed by what felt like an eternal wait for the results, which, in reality, was two days. When I finally received the all-clear, I could breathe again and move on with my life.

Had the test revealed cancer instead of just some abnormal cells, my life would have taken a different trajectory. It's a thought that crosses my mind occasionally. Yet, I believe that what doesn't kill me makes me stronger. Should I ever receive a similar call, I'll breathe through it rather than freeze, taking a more controlled approach to handling the outcome and the results.

I'll pose the necessary questions, seek a clear diagnosis, and avoid feeling like a zombie in limbo, waiting for something to happen.

Being scared doesn't mean we have to shut down or freeze, hoping the problem will resolve itself. Wishing and hoping don't improve situations. Then comes the realization that perhaps there is no answer, or perhaps physically, there's nothing wrong—at least not at a detectable level with today's technology. So, what now? Do you give up?

Or do you keep trying?

Keep searching. Keep doing what you're doing, even if it doesn't have a logical explanation.

What if the diagnosis is that there's genuinely nothing physically wrong with you, and the issues are psychosomatic? Could it be that your mind playing tricks on you—creating symptoms, leading to a disparity between what you perceive and what medical science indicates?

This scenario unfolded for me when I received an unexpected invitation to a dinner hosted by a wellness coach and chiropractor. The timing was serendipitous, arriving just as I was seeking answers, and the event was scheduled for later that week. The topic promised insights into health and wellness, and the lure of a complimentary meal at a new restaurant in town was too good to pass up. The chiropractor proposed that diet and exercise could resolve many health issues, suggesting that reliance on Western medicine and pharmaceuticals might be more harmful than beneficial. Attending the event with an open mind, I hoped to find some guidance, if not a solution, to my ongoing health questions. The dinner took place in a private room at the restaurant, with a select group of attendees. The menu featured exclusively locally sourced, organic, and vegan dishes—a surprising detail, as I hadn't anticipated a vegan setting. After choosing our entrées and settling in with my water, the presentation began. The doctor discussed the impact of diet and exercise on health, emphasizing how many of us could improve our conditions by altering our eating habits and activity levels.

He further clarified that he was a chiropractor certified in nutrition, sharing insights based on his clients' outcomes. He highlighted the issue of overreliance and misuse of drugs developed by Western medicine. According to him, the quest for a quick fix through medication often overshadows the benefits of diet and exercise, leading to a cycle where "wonder drugs" lose their efficacy, and people's health continues to deteriorate.

He advocated for a return to the fundamentals of health, emphasizing the "garbage in, garbage out" principle as much applicable to nutrition as it is to computing. Without consuming wholesome, organic food, the body lacks essential nutrients, resulting in diminished health and vitality. Conversely, proper nutrition supports a robust, energetic lifestyle. His presentation resonated with me, and I immediately signed up for a consultation.

He also recommended involving spouses or partners in the consultation to address any questions they might have about the program. Consequently, I brought my husband along to the appointment. Additionally, he requested copies of any recent blood work or tests to better understand our health backgrounds.

Upon entering the doctor's office, I was immediately struck by the brightness of the white walls. The reception area, nestled in the corner of two glass walls, offered a tranquil view of a retention pond surrounded by exquisite landscaping, creating a serene atmosphere. To the right of the reception, a large room hosted seminars and exercise classes, inviting and warm.

On the left, I found the doctor's office, a space designed to foster a sense of welcome and peace. It felt like an oasis, a supportive environment for anyone on their wellness journey. The doctor reviewed my medical history with a calm demeanor, extending our interview well beyond the scheduled hour and a half, close to two hours.

During our discussion, he addressed my misunderstandings about lab tests and their implications. After thoroughly reviewing my situation, goals, and aspirations, he recommended a six-month program tailored to my needs. While he was uncertain about completely eliminating my tinnitus and vertigo—attributed to hearing loss and the body's response to disparate sounds—he was optimistic about alleviating my headaches and lower back pain through an atlas orthogonal adjustment, a specific chiropractic technique. He even provided a referral to a skilled chiropractor he trusted and had worked with previously.

The doctor mentioned that my headaches and lower back pain could see improvement through an atlas orthogonal adjustment, performed by a skilled chiropractor. He even had a recommendation for me—a professional he had collaborated with during his time as a chiropractor.

The next day, I scheduled an appointment with the atlas orthogonal chiropractor recommended by the doctor. This chiropractor was unlike any I had seen before. Rather than performing general body manipulations, this specialist focused on the head, neck, and shoulders. He began by taking X-rays to ascertain the precise positioning of my bones, then used special software to determine the exact points for adjustment to realign the atlas orthogonal bone in my neck. The thought of having a bone in my neck adjusted was daunting, but my trust in both doctors reassured me to proceed. The experience was astonishing.

Regrettably, the relief was short-lived, necessitating repeat sessions. The chiropractor had cautioned me that, given it had been over 30 years since my car accident, I might need eight to ten treatments for the muscles to relax sufficiently for the adjustment to hold. True to his word, with each visit, the effects of the adjustment extended a bit longer, eventually allowing me to go months between sessions. Then, on the day before Thanksgiving, as I was walking along a neighborhood path, a soccer ball struck me unexpectedly on the right side of my head. The impact was so sudden and forceful that I was surprised I managed to stay on my feet. My husband assisted me back home, where I applied ice to my cheek, hoping to prevent swelling and bruising.

Because the next day was Thanksgiving, no one was around for the holiday, so I had to wait until Friday. Fortunately for me, the chiropractor didn't take two days off for Thanksgiving, and the office was open. I went in and told him my tale of woe. He took an X-ray to confirm what had happened and discovered that I was now 180 degrees out of alignment from my previous adjustment. He was hesitant to make such an extreme adjustment, but then told me he had a similar thing happen to him.

He was doing Tae Kwon Do and took a hit to the head, so he went to get an adjustment. The chiropractor, who was also his mentor, was amazed at the radical change. He did the adjustment, and the situation improved. My doctor was willing to try this new alignment if I was OK with his plan. Given the pain I was in, I would have said yes to just about anything at that point.

He performed the adjustment and asked me to come back in two weeks. Sooner if things didn't improve. I scheduled the appointment for two weeks later. When I came back, he verified everything was holding in place so I could go another month until I came back again. This has been the pattern of our relationship. I enjoyed working with this caring and patient doctor.

He also recommended working with an exercise specialist, who introduced me to simple stretches for my neck and shoulders. Most of these exercises didn't require any equipment, except for one that needed resistance bands. These were exercises I could easily do at home to maintain flexibility and alignment, reducing the likelihood of needing further adjustments. Being limber means your muscles can bend and move as necessary, making them less prone to strain or injury unless subjected to excessive stress. This principle applies broadly.

For example, a tree can bear the weight of snow up to a certain limit. The bough bends under the weight, potentially shaking off the snow if it exceeds the branch's capacity. However, if the branch can no longer bend due to rigidity or excessive weight, it may break. Similarly, if your body isn't properly maintained and kept in optimal condition, it can fail you. A consistent regimen of diet and exercise is crucial for living a long, healthy, and fulfilling life.

Chapter Exercise:

This is a 'doing' exercise rather than a 'thinking and journaling' exercise.

Getting a diagnosis or waiting for a diagnosis can be taxing.

Take some time to let the situation settle in your mind and body.

Then use some relaxation techniques to get in the right frame of mind to deal with the situation.

For example:

Deep breathing

Meditation

Visualizing your perfect day

Chapter Nine
Now what

What do you do when you believe in a higher authority and they let you down? Do you rail against the machine, or pick yourself up and move on with your life? Or do you curl up and give up? Which one are you?

These moments present an opportunity for you to shine. I enjoy what I do and constantly strive to improve myself, seeking the silver lining in every situation. However, I'm not excessively optimistic; those who know me well can attest that I am grounded in reality. I always seek the facts without embellishment. "Just the facts, ma'am," as the saying goes. I don't want any situation to be sugar coated. What do the results show? Whether it's a prognosis of six months to live or an all-clear, I demand the truth. Then, my next question is always about the strategy moving forward. I need to know the next steps.

Improving this situation becomes our focus. Is there a way to make it better, or at least alleviate some of the pain? Identifying who or what can offer assistance is crucial. Does this condition require a specialist's expertise? If so, how do we find them, and what is the earliest appointment available? Are they open to video consultations, or do they strictly offer in-person visits?

Questions about survival rates, the longest survivors, and their unique strategies are also pertinent. Is there documented evidence of what works, and if so, where can it be found? What proactive steps can we take, and is it possible to emulate those who have achieved positive outcomes?

At this point, dwelling on "why me" is counterproductive. Self-pity will not pave the way forward. There must be a purpose for this challenge. Perhaps it's about documenting my journey and spreading awareness, or maybe it's about setting an example for others on how to manage a chronic illness productively.

Why resist making changes that could render life more manageable? Our existence on this planet serves a purpose. Regardless of one's belief in a higher power, the knowledge we acquire and the actions we take hold significance for others.

The essence is that everyone possesses a unique skill or talent—it's all about discovering what that is and then sharing it with the world. Perhaps you excel at writing, or maybe your strength lies in hands-on work. There are those who thrive in investing, while others shine in ideation and innovation. The key is to identify your hidden talent and harness it to its fullest potential. Inventors are meant to invent, writers to write, and artists to create.

We all have skills, both inherent and acquired. It's crucial to leverage these abilities to their maximum. The world should not be deprived of your contributions; your talents should be shared far and wide. It doesn't matter how you view your own abilities; what's important is the joy and enrichment they can bring to others. Remember, significant achievements take time—Rome wasn't built in a day. Michelangelo dedicated years to honing his craft under the tutelage of masters before undertaking the Sistine Chapel.

So, don't give up just yet. You're nearing the finish line, even if you feel lost or uncertain of your next steps. Pause if you must, but don't halt your progress. Reflect deeply on your strengths and consider who might benefit from them.

Consider your potential audience: what do they seek, and what do they require from you? These considerations are vital.

Your gifts are needed by others; they're simply waiting for you to illuminate the path forward.

Chapter Exercise:

Journal for the next fifteen minutes.

Make a list of questions you have about your condition.

Bring the list to your next doctor's appointment.

Ask those questions online to find others in a similar situation. You could find a support group, a YouTube channel, or something similar to help you.

Chapter Ten

It's up to Me

Maybe you are the lucky one—the one who continued searching and discovered a solution to your health issue. Perhaps you encountered that rare medical professional who comprehends your symptoms and offers a strategy for improvement.

It could have been an exercise regimen, a nutritional adjustment, or a comprehensive lifestyle overhaul.

Once you've identified a successful approach, consider creating a club, establishing a Facebook group, writing a book, or proclaiming from the rooftops that you've found an answer. This way, others facing similar challenges will know there's hope and understand they're not alone in their struggles.

Sometimes that is all anyone wants to hear: I am not alone; there are others like me and someone found a way that helped them.

Self-Care

Life may thwart your deepest aspirations due to chronic illness or your responses to it, limiting your choices. Despite the challenges, you've carved out a life for yourself. Whether single or with a family, you may often feel overwhelmed and stressed by your health circumstances.

This situation may necessitate setting aside some "me time." For those burdened with family responsibilities, this could mean planning a solo vacation to escape from everyone and everything, focusing solely on yourself and your desires. It's important to emphasize that neglecting to identify your passion can increase the risk of disrupting your life significantly.

Your inner child, weary of being overlooked, craves attention and fun. Ignoring this need can lead to outcomes that negatively impact not just you but those close to you, potentially ruining long-standing friendships and marriages.

To avoid becoming a cautionary tale, consider taking that solo trip, leaving your cell phone behind. If a getaway isn't feasible, dedicate specific times solely for yourself, turning off your phone to concentrate on your desires and relaxation. Inform others of your availability boundaries, requesting they respect them without inducing guilt.

Use this time to decide what it is you want as well as letting yourself unwind.

Once you've formulated your plan, the next step is to share it with others, detailing your decision and how you envision its implementation. Remember, the retreat allowed you to deeply contemplate and embrace this decision. Your family may need time to match your enthusiasm for the project and the plan, so it's crucial not to be disheartened if they aren't instantly supportive. It's your responsibility to bring them on board by clearly articulating the nature of your plan and its significance to you.

Securing the complete backing of your loved ones is critical; without it, your endeavor might fail, or it could even lead to strain in your marital and family relationships. Success hinges on your ability to effectively communicate your intentions and harmonize your plan with your family life.

The goal is to do what you love while maintaining your relationship with your loved ones. This might demand inventive solutions to ensure responsibilities are managed as you embark on your new project. Embarking on a new venture often means you can't maintain all your current commitments in addition to the new ones. Attempting to juggle too much usually results in stress and may cause either your new venture or your family life to suffer.

If part of the appeal of your new endeavor is to create more time with your family, then prioritize that time. The pursuit of this new venture shouldn't come at the expense of family time. Achieving a balance between work and life is essential for the long-term sustainability of your business or creative project.

Chapter exercise

What does your ideal 'job' look like? Is it a business? A writing career? The sky's the limit. Spend at least fifteen minutes journaling on this question.

Chapter Eleven

Your gifts

For some, your gift is to show courage and grace in the face of unbelievable odds. Others have the ability to continue life after experiencing a significant loss or facing an unexpected illness. While the significance of these gifts may not be immediately apparent to everyone, they manifest in surprising ways. There's much to consider here, but within it all lies a core idea that can guide you from your current position to the next phase of your journey. This path is seldom straightforward; it may twist and turn, ascend and descend, sometimes even circling back on itself.

Upon completing this journey, you'll find yourself at the summit, where the vision might be as breathtaking as witnessing the sunrise over the horizon, an awe-inspiring sight, flawless in every aspect. It might be finding yourself among loved ones who cherish your insights, experiencing a magical moment realized through the acceptance and sharing of your gift. I understand your hesitation to speak about yourself, yet sharing your personal narrative is precisely what your audience needs most.

Your story needs to be heard. Proclaim it for all to hear. Reveal who you are and what you've accomplished. It might feel daunting at first, but the process becomes easier with each telling, and your narrative will grow more polished. Remember, sharing your true experiences is not boastful if it brings value to others.

This underscores the importance of maintaining a clear, vivid vision of what you aspire your future to be—your ideal day, work environment, and client. Keep this vision at the forefront of your mind with every step you take, with every breath. To realize your dream business and make it a source of support for those in need, resilience is key. Prioritize your health through regular exercise, a nutritious diet, and steadily work toward creating that ideal existence.

Maybe you won't get everything you envisioned, but from my experience, you'll find yourself astonishingly close to it. There will be moments along your journey when success seems implausible—that's precisely when you must persevere. It's during these challenging times that you'll encounter the most significant breakthroughs. If you give up now, you'll fall short of reaching the peak, missing out on witnessing a breathtaking sunrise and earning the admiration of many. I believe in you and am confident in your ability to succeed. With belief in yourself and your vision, failure isn't an option.

Everything you've done in your life has brought you to this pivotal moment. You stand before a door; you can either choose to step through it or remain immobilized by fear, yearning for change. Once you've glimpsed the light, it becomes impossible to ignore. Don't hesitate—start today. You are deserving. You are capable. Now is your time to shine.

My own medical challenges could have restricted my options, yet I chose to confront pain and uncertainty, leading to success in my endeavors. Despite initial doubts about accepting my first job, starting a business, or writing this book, I never regretted embarking on these ventures. However, I do harbor some regrets about opportunities I passed up due to concerns that my health issues might interfere.

You might wonder, "Is such success feasible for me, starting from where I am?" While some may view any change as beneficial, you recognize that you cannot continue on a path marked by constant illness and fatigue. Opting to modify your diet is a step towards potential improvement. Investigate various nutritional plans to find one that suits your specific needs. The Mediterranean and migraine diets were particularly effective for me; perhaps starting with these could positively impact your symptoms, considering any allergies or food preferences you have. There might be a suitable path for you too.

For this to work, you need to be excited to get started *today.* You want to feel better. You want to look better. Many of you have been thinking about this extensively and for too long. It remains to be seen if you can pull it off. However, things will never change if you don't change something.

Are you committed? Are you willing to change your mindset and decide not to spend one more day feeling sorry for yourself?

Chapter Exercise

Journal for about fifteen minutes.

Make a list of things you would like to change in your life.

Make a list of things you would love to do, regardless of what it costs.

What are you willing to do today to change your current situation?

Chapter Twelve
A new beginning

This book is about a woman's journey. Though the protagonist is named Josette, it could just as easily be your name, or that of someone you know. It's a narrative that could mirror your own path, marked by trials and tribulations, set against the backdrop of launching a business, authoring a book, or embarking on a creative project.

What is the right thing to do when I have this mystery illness and don't always feel 100 percent? Can I be successful if I suffer a migraine and have to cancel a client session?

How do I handle physical and mental challenges when they come up?

What is right for me?

Have I done all I can?

How do I find the right mentor?

Can I use this book to its full advantage and really change my life?

What does the perfect day look like for me? The concept of achieving financial freedom tantalizes me, enticing me to believe in its possibility. Yet, as I delve deeper into the thought, it appears increasingly elusive.

The myriad considerations begin to merge, forming a complex web that seems insurmountable. How can I do this alone? What makes me think that someone like me can emulate Josette's path to transformation?

This moment signifies the end of the former you and heralds the arrival of a new version. You've navigated through adversity, sought out specialists for your medical issues, and taken the bold step of launching your business, writing your book, or pursuing your passion project.

Your well-being has improved significantly, surprising even the skeptics around you. Your book is on the verge of being published, your business has attracted paying clients and is yielding profits. The skeptics in your life remain mired in their pessimism, now tinged with envy at your accomplishments.

They rationalize, "She succeeded because she doesn't have children," or "That health issue wasn't as serious as she made it out to be. Look at everything she's managed to do. She must have been exaggerating." Or even, "Her business idea, her book, her venture—they're all so basic. Her clients must not know better. I wish I had pursued that. Actually, it was my idea. She just executed what I had suggested."

You need to tune out these negative influences. Sometimes, you may need to 'unfriend' them entirely, in both the online and offline worlds. Only you know how much their negative influence is affecting you and whether you can continue to associate with them or need to remove them from your life. Such comments reflect their inability to appreciate the effort and resilience required to transform one's life. They underscore a fundamental truth: success often breeds criticism, especially from those who have yet to dare as you have.

It is unpleasant when this happens, especially if you've been friends for a long time. But remember how you used to feel versus where you are now, and ask yourself this question:

Do I want to be dragged back to that point in time in my life?

Or do I prefer how my life is going now?

For some of you, this will be a simple choice. Others still think that with enough time and effort you can get your friend to move from negativity island to positivity paradise. Most negative influencers can't be swayed. They are so stuck in their own fear that no matter what you say or do, they will always have some excuse why things are different for you.

Why are you so lucky? That's what they want to know. And what you should know is it is your decision to remove them from your life. You'll know when the time is right, just like you knew when to implement this new strategy for your life.

As you implement changes in your lifestyle, diet, exercise habits, and pursue new ventures like your book or business, you're witnessing substantial improvements in your life. You're becoming healthier and more robust with each passing day.

Your journey has garnered a following, including many who you've never met, all rooting for your success. They are inspired by your message and aspire to achieve their own dream lives through the wisdom you share. Your enthusiastic supporters are eager to witness your continued growth and to evolve alongside you.

When doubts about your decisions surface, and you're contemplating your next steps, keep this vision of support and progress at the forefront of your mind. This guidance might extend to your personal relationships as well. Any partnership where one person heavily relies on the other can face challenges, especially if you begin to alter that dynamic. A sudden shift might leave your spouse feeling uncertain or fearful that you're drifting away, so it's crucial to make them feel a part of your journey. In some cases, you might find that your partner prefers to maintain control and might resist your moves toward independence. These are personal dilemmas you'll need to navigate and resolve.

I cannot tell you the right path for you to take. I do want you to succeed and step into your dream life.

"Help me be aware of my limitations and my strengths."

This is my mantra to keep moving forward every day.

The answer is simple. This book challenges the assumption that simple and obvious topics are truly simple or obvious.

Some people can spend a minute looking at one of those old 'magic-eye' pictures and be able to see a clown or a giraffe or whatever is behind what looks like abstract art or dots on a page. Others can look at that same artwork for hours and see nothing except a multicolored abstract art piece.

This book is the same. No two people will have the same outcome or the same conclusion.

It is magic. The magic of being in the right place at the right time and open to the mysteries of the universe.

About the Author

JOSETTE MANDELA, an MBA-trained author, specializes in empowering women by teaching them fundamental financial skills.

Before embarking on a transformative health journey, Josette worked as a consultant for various financial institutions, where she enjoyed lucrative earnings but faced constant uncertainty regarding job security.

Her career trajectory took a significant turn following an ear infection that led to vertigo and tinnitus, prompting her to perceive these challenges as a universal sign to reassess her life's direction.

Motivated by this revelation, Josette embraced her true calling: writing and establishing a business centered on educating women about financial literacy. This endeavor led to the creation of her second book, a project that seemed to demand its own existence. Josette realized her mission extended beyond financial education. Recognizing that many women were hindered by health issues that also impacted their financial stability, she dedicated herself to addressing both facets, aiming to liberate women from the constraints of poor health and financial insecurity.

Josette can be found at https://josettemandela.com or on Facebook at https://www.facebook.com/TheMoneyGirlonTwitter.

Other books by this author: *Woman's Guide to Money Freedom, Saving, Investing and Building Wealth for Beginners.*

If you enjoyed this book, please remember to leave a review on Amazon.

If you haven't done so already, don't forget to grab your bonus materials.

To download the free bonus material for this book please visit:

https://www.TheResilienceResetBook.com/bonus

There you will find useful tips to help you on your journey.

www.ingramcontent.com/pod-product-compliance
Lightning Source LLC
Chambersburg PA
CBHW031202020426
42333CB00013B/777